Ketogenic Diet Cookbook for Women over 50

-Feel 35 Again with Anti - Inflammatory Recipes to Lose Belly Fat and Increase Your Energy -

[Dr. Dean Chasey]

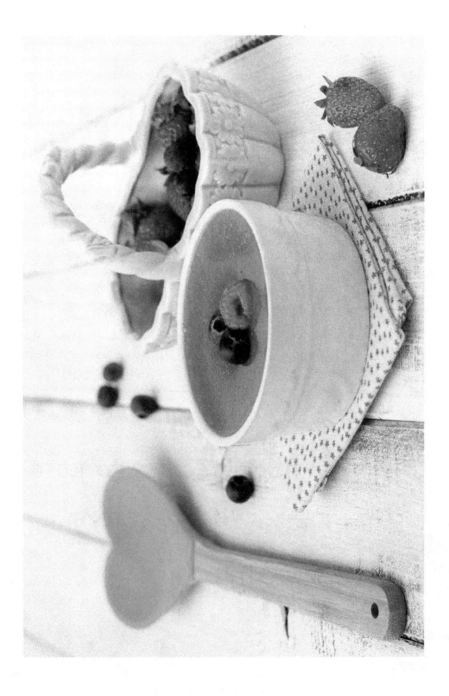

Table Of Content

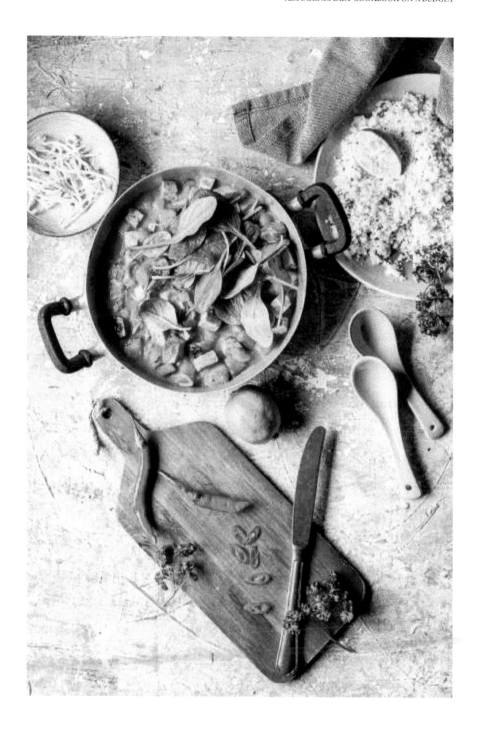

The following Book is reproduced below with the goal of providing information that is as accurate and reliable as possible. Regardless, purchasing this Book can be seen as consent to the fact that both the publisher and the author of this book are in no way experts on the topics discussed within and that any recommendations or suggestions that are made herein are for entertainment purposes only. Professionals should be consulted as needed prior to undertaking any of the action endorsed herein.

This declaration is deemed fair and valid by both the American Bar Association and the Committee of Publishers Association and is legally binding throughout the United States.

Furthermore, the transmission, duplication, or reproduction of any of the following work including specific information will be considered an illegal act irrespective of if it is done electronically or in print. This extends to creating a secondary or tertiary copy of the work or a recorded copy and is only allowed with the express written consent from the Publisher. All additional right reserved.

The information in the following pages is broadly considered a truthful and accurate account of facts and as such, any inattention, use, or misuse of the information in question by the reader will render any resulting actions solely under their purview. There are no scenarios in which the publisher or the original author of this work can be in any fashion deemed liable for any hardship or damages that may befall them after undertaking information described herein.

Additionally, the information in the following pages is intended only for informational purposes and should thus be thought of as universal. As befitting its nature, it is presented without assurance regarding its prolonged validity or interim quality. Trademarks that are mentioned are done without written consent and can in no way be considered an endorsement from the trademark holder.

CHAPTER 1: **BREAKFAST**

Bacon & Blue Cheese Cup

Prep:

10 mins

Additional:

1 hr

Total:

1 hr 10 mins

Servings:

10

Yield:

10 servings

Ingredients

½ cup blue cheese salad dressing
1 (2.5 ounce) package cooked real bacon pieces (such as Hormel™)
½ cup mayonnaise
1 (16 ounce) bag coleslaw mix
1 cup quartered cherry tomatoes
salt and pepper to taste

Directions

1

Combine mayonnaise, salad dressing, salt, and pepper in a large bowl.
Stir in the coleslaw mix and bacon. Add the tomatoes, and toss gently.
Cover, and refrigerate for 1 hour or overnight before serving.

Nutrition

Per Serving: 205 calories; protein 4.5g; carbohydrates 7.6g; fat 17.9g; cholesterol 15mg; sodium 434.6mg.

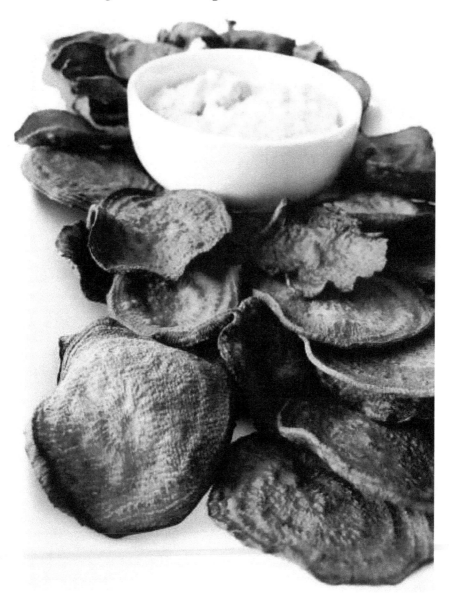

Avocado and Feta Egg White Omelet

Prep:

5 mins

Cook:

5 mins

Total:

10 mins

Servings:

1

Yield:

1 omelet

Ingredients

½ cup egg whites

1 teaspoon paprika

3 leaves fresh basil

½ avocado, sliced

½ tablespoon olive oil

Directions

1

Mix egg whites and paprika together in a bowl.

2

Heat olive oil in a small skillet over medium heat. Pour in egg white mixture; cook for 1 minute. Place basil leaves over egg whites. Cook until egg white starts to firm up, about 1 minute. Spread avocado on top and sprinkle with feta cheese. Cook for 3 minutes more. Fold in half to form the omelet.

Nutrition

Per Serving: 336 calories; protein 18.3g; carbohydrates 11.5g; fat 25.8g; cholesterol 16.8mg; sodium 420.7mg.

Keto Breakfast Frittata

Prep:

10 mins

Cook:

30 mins

Additional:

5 mins

Total:

45 mins

Servings:

6

Yield:

1 12-inch frittata

Ingredients

4 ounces bulk breakfast sausage

8 eggs

½ cup chopped onion

salt and ground black pepper to taste

2 tablespoons heavy cream

2 tablespoons butter

1 cup chopped mushrooms

1 cup shredded Cheddar cheese

⅔ cup chopped red bell pepper

8 drops hot pepper sauce (such as Tabasco®)

½ cup chopped fresh spinach

Directions

1

Preheat the oven to 325 degrees F.

2

Crumble sausage into a 12-inch nonstick, oven-proof skillet over medium heat. Cook until browned, about 4 minutes.

3

Meanwhile, whisk eggs in a large bowl. Add cream and hot pepper sauce; mix well.

4

Add butter to the skillet with browned sausage and melt around the inside rim of the skillet. Add mushrooms, red bell pepper, onion, salt, and pepper. Cook until onion is soft and translucent, about 4 minutes. Turn off heat and stir in spinach. Cook for 1 minute in hot skillet, then sprinkle with Cheddar cheese. Pour egg mixture on top, making sure all the Ingredients are submerged.

5

Place skillet in the preheated oven and bake until eggs are set and no longer jiggle, about 20 minutes. Remove from oven and allow to sit for 1 to 2 minutes, before cutting into serving pieces.

Nutrition

Per Serving: 283 calories; protein 16.5g; carbohydrates 3.8g; fat 22.7g; cholesterol 295.4mg; sodium 443mg.

Smoked Salmon Dill Eggs Benedict

Prep:

10 mins

Cook:

10 mins

Total:

20 mins

Servings:

2

Yield:

2 servings

Ingredients

¼ cup butter, softened
2 tablespoons fresh dill
1 pinch cayenne pepper
salt and ground black pepper to taste
1 teaspoon white vinegar
1 teaspoon lemon zest
1 pinch salt
4 eggs
4 ounces sliced smoked salmon
1 pinch cayenne pepper
salt and ground black pepper to taste
2 English muffins, split and toasted
4 small fresh dill sprigs

Directions

1

Stir butter, dill, lemon zest, cayenne pepper, salt, and black pepper in a bowl until combined. Set aside.

2

Fill a large saucepan with 2 to 3 inches of water and bring to a boil over high heat. Reduce heat to medium-low, pour in vinegar and a pinch of salt. Crack an egg into a bowl then gently slip the egg into the water. Repeat with remaining eggs. Poach eggs until whites are firm and yolks have thickened but are not hard, 4 to 6 minutes. Remove eggs from water with a slotted spoon, dab on a kitchen towel to remove excess water, then transfer to a warm plate.

3

Generously spread each English muffin half with dill butter. Top with a layer of smoked salmon, then 1 poached egg. Season with cayenne pepper, salt, and black pepper to taste. Garnish with a dill sprig and serve.

Nutrition

Per Serving: 528 calories; protein 26.3g; carbohydrates 27g; fat 35.3g; cholesterol 399.6mg; sodium 1297.7mg.

Cream and Raspberries topping

Prep:

5 mins

Cook:

15 mins

Total:

20 mins

Servings:

12

Yield:

3 cups

Ingredients

1 ½ cups frozen raspberries

½ cup white sugar

¼ cup water

1 cup frozen blueberries

Directions

1

Combine the raspberries, blueberries, sugar, and water in a small saucepan; bring to a boil and cook at a boil for 5 minutes, scraping the bottom as needed to keep from burning. Reduce heat to low; simmer the mixture until thick, about 10 minutes. Serve warm.

Nutrition

Per Serving: 47 calories; protein 0.2g; carbohydrates 11.9g; fat 0.1g; sodium 0.3mg.

Pork Casserole

Prep:

15 mins

Cook:

1 hr

Total:

1 hr 15 mins

Servings:

4

Yield:

4 servings

Ingredients

4 pork chops, well trimmed

½ cup raisins

1 (10.75 ounce) can condensed oxtail soup

⅓ cup water

1 large cooking apple, peeled, cored and chopped

Directions

1

Preheat the oven to 350 degrees F. Place the pork chops into a buttered 9x13 inch baking dish. Add the apple and raisins. Pour the soup and water into a small bowl, and mix together. Pour the soup over the pork chops.

2

Bake, covered, in the preheated oven until the pork chops are fully cooked, about 1 hour.

Nutrition

Per Serving: 552 calories; protein 36.6g; carbohydrates 60.2g; fat 18.4g; cholesterol 87.2mg; sodium 4988.2mg.

Ciabatta Bread

Prep:

30 mins

Cook:

25 mins

Additional:

1 hr

Total:

1 hr 55 mins

Servings:

24

Yield:

2 loaves

Ingredients

1 ½ cups water

1 teaspoon white sugar

1 tablespoon olive oil

3 ¼ cups bread flour

1 ½ teaspoons bread machine yeast

1 ½ teaspoons salt

Directions

1

Place Ingredients into the pan of the bread machine in the order suggested by the manufacturer. Select the Dough cycle, and Start. (See Editor's Note for stand mixer instructions.)

2

Dough will be quite sticky and wet once cycle is completed; resist the temptation to add more flour. Place dough on a generously floured board, cover with a large bowl or greased plastic wrap, and let rest for 15 minutes.

3

Lightly flour baking sheets or line them with parchment paper. Using a serrated knife, divide dough into 2 pieces, and form each into a 3x14-inch oval. Place loaves on prepared sheets and dust lightly with flour. Cover, and let rise in a draft-free place for approximately 45 minutes.

4

Preheat oven to 425 degrees F.

5

Spritz loaves with water. Place loaves in the oven, positioned on the middle rack. Bake until golden brown, 25 to 30 minutes.

Nutrition

Per Serving: 73 calories; protein 2.3g; carbohydrates 13.7g; fat 0.9g; sodium 146.3mg.

Tofu Scramble

Prep:

10 mins

Cook:

15 mins

Total:

25 mins

Servings:

4

Yield:

4 servings

Ingredients

1 tablespoon olive oil

1 (14.5 ounce) can peeled and diced tomatoes with juice

1 bunch green onions, chopped

1 (12 ounce) package firm silken tofu, drained and mashed

ground turmeric to taste

salt and pepper to taste

Directions

1

Heat olive oil in a medium skillet over medium heat, and saute green onions until tender. Stir in tomatoes with juice and mashed tofu.

Season with salt, pepper, and turmeric. Reduce heat, and simmer until heated through. Sprinkle with Cheddar cheese to serve.

Nutrition

Per Serving: 190 calories; protein 12g; carbohydrates 9.7g; fat 11.5g; cholesterol 18.1mg; sodium 305.8mg.

Cheeseburger Pie

Prep:

15 mins

Cook:

30 mins

Total:

45 mins

Servings:

6

Yield:

6 servings

Ingredients

1 pound lean (at least 80%) ground beef

1 cup milk

1 medium onion, chopped

⅛ teaspoon pepper

1 cup shredded Cheddar cheese

½ cup Bisquick™ Gluten Free mix

½ teaspoon salt

3 eggs

Directions

1

Heat oven to 400 degrees F. Spray 9-inch glass pie plate with cooking spray. In 10-inch skillet, cook beef and onion over medium-high heat, stirring frequently, until beef is thoroughly cooked; drain. Stir in salt and pepper. Spread in pie plate; sprinkle with cheese.

2

In medium bowl, stir Bisquick mix, milk and eggs until blended. Pour into pie plate.

3

Bake 25 to 30 minutes or until knife inserted in center comes out clean.

Nutrition

Per Serving: 319 calories; protein 24.3g; carbohydrates 11.8g; fat 18.9g; cholesterol 165.6mg; sodium 493.6mg.

Coated Shrimp

Prep:

15 mins

Cook:

15 mins

Total:

30 mins

Servings:

4

Yield:

4 servings

Ingredients

1 cup all-purpose flour

1 pound uncooked medium shrimp, peeled and deveined

⅔ cup beer

½ teaspoon salt

2 cups sweetened flaked coconut

1 cup vegetable oil for frying

1 large egg

Directions

1

Beat flour, beer, egg, and salt in a bowl with an electric mixer on low until batter is smooth. Spread coconut flakes in a shallow dish.

2

Dip shrimp into beer batter, shaking off excess, then press into coconut. Place shrimp onto a plate while breading the rest; do not stack.

3

Heat vegetable oil in a skillet over medium-high heat until hot but not smoking, 3 to 4 minutes. Fry about a third of the shrimp in the hot oil until golden brown, 2 to 3 minutes. Allow shrimp to drain on a wire rack set over paper towels. Repeat with remaining shrimp.

Nutrition

Per Serving: 581 calories; protein 25.1g; carbohydrates 54.8g; fat 28.3g; cholesterol 203.1mg; sodium 720.4mg.

CHAPTER 2: SOUPS & SALADS

Salsa Verde Chicken and Rice Tortilla Soup

Prep:

5 mins

Cook:

12 mins

Total:

17 mins

Servings:

4

Yield:

4 servings

Ingredients

4 cups water

2 cooked chicken breast halves, shredded

1 cup red bell pepper, diced

1 (5.4 ounce) package Knorr® Fiesta Sides™ - Mexican Rice

1 cup salsa verde

½ lime, juiced

Directions

1

Measure water into a pot and bring to a boil over medium-high heat. Add chicken, Knorr® Fiesta SidesTM - Mexican Rice, red bell pepper, and salsa verde. Reduce to a low and simmer until the rice is fully cooked, about 10 minutes. Stir in lime juice, continue to simmer for another 2 minutes.

2

Serve in bowls topped with crushed tortilla chips.

Nutrition

Per Serving: 411 calories; protein 35g; carbohydrates 21.3g; fat 10.9g; cholesterol 82.5mg; sodium 328.2mg.

Mini Cobb Salad with Avocado Dressing

Prep:

35 mins

Total:

35 mins

Servings:

4

Yield:

4 servings

Ingredients

Avocado Dressing:

½ lemon, juiced

1 clove garlic, minced

½ teaspoon ground cumin

¼ teaspoon salt

Dash cayenne pepper

2 tablespoons olive oil

¼ cup water

1 small ripe avocado - peeled, pitted, and diced

Salad:

6 cups coarsely chopped salad greens (iceberg, romaine, etc.)

4 slices turkey-style bacon, cooked and chopped

2 tomatoes, cut into wedges

2 cups diced cooked chicken

½ cup thinly sliced red onion

2 ounces blue cheese, crumbled

4 hard-cooked eggs, peeled and coarsely chopped

Directions

1

Avocado Dressing: In a blender or mini-chopper, blend avocado, oil, lemon juice, garlic, cumin, salt, cayenne pepper and water, until smooth. Thin dressing with additional water if desired.

2

Salad: Divide salad greens among individual plates. Place a mound of chicken in center of each. Arrange turkey-style bacon, tomatoes, egg wedges and red onion around chicken. Sprinkle with blue cheese. Drizzle with dressing just before serving.

Nutrition

Per Serving: 474 calories; protein 32.9g; carbohydrates 11.7g; fat 33.8g; cholesterol 265.3mg; sodium 687.6mg.

Chilled Tomato & Avocado Soup

Prep:

20 mins

Additional:

2 hrs

Total:

2 hrs 20 mins

Servings:

6

Yield:

6 servings

Ingredients

1 ripe tomato, peeled and quartered

cayenne pepper to taste

2 large avocados - peeled, pitted, and sliced

1 small onion, quartered

¼ cup fresh lemon juice

1 quart tomato juice

1 ¼ cups plain nonfat yogurt

salt to taste

¼ cup chopped fresh chives

1 green bell pepper, chopped

Directions

1

Place tomato, avocados, onion, green bell pepper, and lemon juice into the bowl of a food processor, and process until smooth. Pour in 1 cup tomato juice, and process to blend.

2

Transfer mixture to a large bowl, and mix in remaining tomato juice and 1 cup yogurt. Season to taste with salt. Chill for 2 hours.

3

Serve in bowls garnished with dollops of yogurt, chives, and a sprinkling of cayenne pepper.

Nutrition

Per Serving: 215 calories; protein 5.8g; carbohydrates 22.7g; fat 14.1g; cholesterol 1mg; sodium 663.8mg.

CHAPTER 3: LUNCH

Keto Lasagna

Prep:

10 mins

Cook:

40 mins

Additional:

10 mins

Total:

1 hr

Servings:

4

Yield:

1 8x8-inch lasagna

Ingredients

1 pound lean ground beef

½ cup shredded Parmesan cheese

½ teaspoon salt

1 tablespoon avocado oil

½ cup minced onion

1 teaspoon minced garlic

1 ½ cups marinara sauce

½ teaspoon ground black pepper

½ cup ricotta cheese, drained

1 ½ cups shredded mozzarella cheese

1 large egg

Directions

1

Preheat the oven to 400 degrees F.

2

Add ground beef to a skillet and season with salt and pepper. Cook and stir beef over medium-high heat until browned and crumbled, about 10 minutes. Remove to a strainer and set aside. Pour oil into the same skillet and heat over medium heat. Add onion and cook until soft and translucent, 4 to 6 minutes. Add garlic and cook until fragrant, about 30 seconds.

3

Return beef to the skillet. Pour in marinara sauce, mix to combine, and turn off the heat.

4

Mix ricotta cheese, Parmesan cheese, 1/2 cup mozzarella cheese, and egg together in a bowl. Place the meat mixture in an 8x8-inch oven-safe casserole dish. Spread the cheese mixture over the meat and sprinkle with remaining 1 cup mozzarella cheese.

5

Bake until casserole is golden brown and cheese is melted, 20 to 25 minutes. Let rest 10 minutes before serving

Nutritions

Per Serving: 479 calories; protein 38.9g; carbohydrates 11.7g; fat 30.1g; cholesterol 156.8mg; sodium 1178.7mg.

Afritada Chicken

Prep:

40 mins

Cook:

48 mins

Total:

1 hr 28 mins

Servings:

6

Yield:

6 servings

Ingredients

1 tablespoon vegetable oil

3 cloves garlic, crushed and chopped

1 cup seeded and chopped tomatoes

1 (3 pound) whole chicken, cut into pieces

3 cups water

3 potatoes, quartered

1 onion, chopped

1 carrot, chopped

salt and ground black pepper to taste

1 green bell pepper, seeded and cut into matchsticks

Directions

1

Heat oil in a large wok over medium heat; add garlic. Cook and stir until fragrant, about 3 minutes. Add onion; cook and stir until translucent, about 5 minutes. Stir in tomatoes; cook, mashing with a fork, until flesh and skin separate, about 5 minutes.

2

Place chicken in the wok; cook and stir until lightly browned, about 5 minutes. Pour in water. Cover and bring to a boil. Stir in tomato sauce; simmer until flavors combine, about 15 minutes.

3

Mix potatoes into the wok; simmer until tender, about 10 minutes. Stir in bell pepper and carrot; simmer until softened, about 5 minutes. Season with salt and pepper.

Nutritions

Per Serving: 594 calories; protein 22.8g; carbohydrates 25.1g; fat 44.7g; cholesterol 80.3mg; sodium 324.2mg.

Chicken Enchiladas

Prep:

15 mins

Cook:

20 mins

Total:

35 mins

Servings:

8

Yield:

8 enchiladas

Ingredients

cooking spray

1 cup chunky salsa

6 ounces cream cheese, softened

8 (8 inch) flour tortillas

1 (15 ounce) can enchilada sauce

3 cups shredded, cooked chicken

½ cup shredded Mexican cheese blend

Directions

1

Preheat the oven to 375 degrees F. Line a rimmed baking sheet with aluminum foil, then spray with cooking spray.

2

Combine salsa and cream cheese in a large pan over medium heat; cook and stir until cream cheese has melted and mixture is creamy and thoroughly combined, 3 to 5 minutes. Add chicken and cook until heated through, 2 to 3 minutes.

3

Spoon chicken mixture into tortillas and roll into enchiladas. Place, seam-side down, on the prepared baking sheet. Top with enchilada sauce.

4

Bake in the preheated oven for 10 minutes. Top with Mexican cheese. Bake until cheese is melted, 6 to 10 minutes more. Serve hot.

Nutritions

Per Serving: 409 calories; protein 21.6g; carbohydrates 33.7g; fat 20.6g; cholesterol 70.6mg; sodium 706.2mg.

Crunchy Taco Chicken Wings

Servings:

3

Yield:

2 to 4 servings

Ingredients

1 (16 ounce) package chicken drumettes

2 cups crushed tortilla chip crumbs

1 (1.25 ounce) package taco seasoning mix

Directions

1

Preheat oven to 350 degrees F.

2

Rinse chicken pieces and pat dry. In a shallow dish or bowl, mix together the taco seasoning mix and tortilla chip crumbs.

3

Roll chicken pieces in chip mixture and place coated chicken in a lightly greased 9x13 inch baking dish. Bake in the preheated oven for 20 minutes. Turn chicken pieces and bake for another 15 to 20 minutes.

Nutritions

Per Serving: 461 calories; protein 29.1g; carbohydrates 19.4g; fat 28.2g; cholesterol 116.5mg; sodium 1045.9mg.

Keto Beef Burgers

Prep:

15 mins

Cook:

20 mins

Additional:

20 mins

Total:

55 mins

Servings:

8

Yield:

8 burgers

Ingredients

2 pounds ground beef
1 onion, chopped
½ teaspoon ground black pepper
3 cloves garlic, minced
1 teaspoon Italian seasoning
1 teaspoon salt
1 (8 ounce) package mushrooms, chopped
cooking spray

Directions

1

Remove ground beef from the refrigerator; let stand at room temperature for 20 minutes.

2

Mix mushrooms, onion, garlic, Italian seasoning, salt, and pepper together in a large bowl. Mix in beef. Form beef mixture into 1/2-inch-thick patties.

3

Grease an indoor grill pan with cooking spray. Cook patties in batches until browned and no longer pink in the center, about 10 minutes per side.

Nutritions

Per Serving: 216 calories; protein 20.1g; carbohydrates 2.8g; fat 13.5g; cholesterol 68.8mg; sodium 358.2mg.

Saucy Slow Cooker Pork Chops

Prep:

15 mins

Cook:

6 hrs 10 mins

Total:

6 hrs 25 mins

Servings:

5

Yield:

5 servings

Ingredients

3 tablespoons olive oil

1 (8 ounce) can tomato sauce

1 onion, sliced

2 green bell peppers, sliced

¼ cup brown sugar

1 tablespoon apple cider vinegar

2 teaspoons Worcestershire sauce

5 boneless pork chops, trimmed

1 ½ teaspoons salt

Directions

1

Heat olive oil in a large skillet over medium heat; cook pork chops in the hot oil until browned, about 5 minutes per side. Transfer browned pork chops to a slow cooker; top pork chops with onion and green peppers.

2

Whisk tomato sauce, brown sugar, vinegar, Worcestershire sauce, and salt together in a bowl. Pour sauce into slow cooker, gently stirring to coat meat and vegetables.

3

Cook pork chops on Low until tender, 6 to 8 hours.

4

Transfer pork chops to a serving platter; tent with aluminum foil to keep warm. Whisk cornstarch into sauce until thickened; spoon sauce and vegetables over pork chops.

Nutritions

Per Serving: 321 calories; protein 24.8g; carbohydrates 20.9g; fat 15.2g; cholesterol 59.1mg; sodium 994.6mg.

Maiale al Latte

Prep:

15 mins

Cook:

1 hr 35 mins

Total:

1 hr 50 mins

Servings:

4

Yield:

4 servings

Ingredients

1 tablespoon olive oil

2 slices bacon, coarsely chopped

salt and freshly ground black pepper to taste

1 small yellow onion, diced

4 cloves garlic, sliced

1 ¼ cups chicken broth

½ cup creme fraiche

1 ½ pounds pork shoulder, cut into 2-inch chunks

2 tablespoons chopped fresh sage leaves

¼ cup olive oil

15 whole fresh sage leaves

1 pinch red pepper flakes

Directions

1

Pour 1 tablespoon olive oil into a skillet, place over medium heat, and cook bacon, stirring often, until crisp and bacon fat has rendered into the skillet, about 5 minutes.

2

Season pork cubes generously with salt and black pepper. Remove bacon from pan and set aside, reserving fat in pan. Turn heat to medium-high and brown pork pieces in bacon drippings until well browned on both sides, about 5 minutes per side. Transfer meat to a bowl, leaving pan drippings in skillet.

3

Turn heat to medium and stir in chopped onion and a pinch of salt. Cook and stir onion until translucent and slightly browned, about 5 minutes. Stir garlic into onion and cook until fragrant, about 1 minute.

4

Pour chicken broth and creme fraiche into onion mixture; whisk until smooth. Scrape up and dissolve any browned bits of food on the bottom of the skillet. Bring mixture to a simmer.

5

Return bacon to sauce and stir in 2 tablespoons chopped sage. Place pork pieces into simmering sauce along with any accumulated juices from the meat. Reduce heat to low, cover, and simmer until meat is almost tender, about 1 hour.

6

Raise heat to medium and cook uncovered until pan sauce reduces and thickens and meat is very tender, about 20 more minutes. Stir red pepper flakes into sauce; adjust seasonings to taste.

7

Heat 1/4 cup olive oil in a small skillet over medium heat; drop whole sage leaves into the hot oil and cook, lightly tossing leaves in the oil, until crisp, about 15 seconds. Drain sage leaves on paper towels and crumble over pork.

Nutritions

Per Serving: 514 calories; protein 20.9g; carbohydrates 4.7g; fat 46.2g; cholesterol 114.4mg; sodium 568.8mg.

Vegetable Casserole with Eggplant

Prep:

20 mins

Cook:

50 mins

Total:

1 hr 10 mins

Servings:

6

Yield:

6 servings

Ingredients

1 large eggplant, peeled and diced

3 tablespoons butter

6 ounces grated sharp Cheddar cheese

3 tablespoons flour

1 green bell pepper, chopped

1 medium onion, chopped

2 tablespoons brown sugar, or more to taste

1 teaspoon salt

1 (28 ounce) can stewed tomatoes

⅓ cup fine bread crumbs

Directions

1

Preheat the oven to 350 degrees F.

2

Bring a large saucepan of water to a boil. Add eggplant and cook until tender, 10 to 15 minutes. Drain and pour eggplant into an 8-inch square baking dish.

3

Melt butter in a 3-quart saucepan on medium heat. Add flour and mix to create a paste. Add tomatoes, bell pepper, onion, brown sugar, and salt and cook over medium to medium-high heat. Stir occasionally until mixture bubbles and thickens, 5 to 10 minutes. Pour mixture over the eggplant in the baking dish.

4

Cover the vegetables in the baking dish with Cheddar cheese and bread crumbs.

5

Bake in the preheated oven until hot and bubbly, 30 to 40 minutes.

Nutritions

Per Serving: 281 calories; protein 10.9g; carbohydrates 26.4g; fat 15.9g; cholesterol 45mg; sodium 840.2mg.

Bacon Stuffed Avocados

Prep:

10 mins

Cook:

20 mins

Total:

30 mins

Servings:

8

Yield:

8 avocado halves

Ingredients

8 slices bacon
2 cloves garlic, chopped
½ cup butter
¼ cup red wine vinegar
1 tablespoon soy sauce
salt to taste
4 avocados - halved, pitted, and peeled
¼ cup brown sugar

Directions

1

Place bacon in a large skillet and cook over medium-high heat, turning occasionally, until evenly browned, about 10 – 12 minutes. Drain bacon slices on paper towels; crumble.

2

Mix butter, brown sugar, vinegar, soy sauce, and garlic in a saucepan; cook and stir mixture over medium heat until sugar is dissolved, about 10 minutes.

3

Sprinkle avocado halves with salt; fill each half with crumbled bacon. Drizzle sauce over filled avocados.

Nutritions

Per Serving: 333 calories; protein 5.7g; carbohydrates 14.1g; fat 30.1g; cholesterol 40.5mg; sodium 413.7mg.

Parchment Baked Salmon

Prep:

15 mins

Cook:

25 mins

Total:

40 mins

Servings:

2

Yield:

2 servings

Ingredients

1 (8 ounce) salmon fillet

1 lemon, thinly sliced

¼ cup chopped basil leaves

olive oil cooking spray

salt and ground black pepper to taste

Directions

1

Place an oven rack in the lowest position in oven and preheat oven to 400 degrees F.

2

Place salmon fillet with skin side down in the middle of a large piece of parchment paper; season with salt and black pepper. Cut 2 3-inch slits into the fish with a sharp knife. Stuff chopped basil leaves into the slits. Spray fillet with cooking spray and arrange lemon slices on top.

3

Fold edges of parchment paper over the fish several times to seal into an airtight packet. Place sealed packet onto a baking sheet.

4

Bake fish on the bottom rack of oven until salmon flakes easily and meat is pink and opaque with an interior of slightly darker pink color, about 25 minutes. An instant-read meat thermometer inserted into the thickest part of the fillet should read at least 145 degrees F. To serve, cut the parchment paper open and remove lemon slices before plating fish.

Nutritions

Per Serving: 175 calories; protein 24.8g; carbohydrates 6.1g; fat 6.9g; cholesterol 49.9mg; sodium 48.3mg

CHAPTER 4: **DINNER**

Lamb Shashlyk

Prep:

15 mins

Cook:

12 mins

Total:

27 mins

Servings:

3 to 4 servings

Ingredients

1 pound lamb trimmed of all fat, and cut into 2" cubes (leg or shoulder of lamb)

1/2 cup lemon juice

1/2 cup olive oil

1 teaspoon black pepper

1 teaspoon salt

1/4 teaspoon ground red pepper

2 medium onions (cut into eighths)

1-pint cherry tomatoes

2 large green peppers (cut into 1-inch chunks)

  s to Make It

In a bowl, combine lamb, olive oil, lemon juice, pepper, salt, and red pepper. Allow to marinate at least 2 to 3 hours prior to cooking.

Place marinated beef on skewers (about 6 cubes per skewer). Be sure to apply a light coat of oil on the skewer prior to threading the meat.

Place vegetables on separate skewers, alternating type of vegetable. The meat and veggies are cooked on different skewers because the meat will take longer to grill.

Cook lamb shashlik skewers on the grill or under the broiler for 10 to 12 minutes, or until desired doneness. Turn to ensure even cooking.

Grill vegetable skewers for last 5 minutes of grilling. Turn. The vegetables should be crisp, yet tender. Be careful not to overcook.

Mango-Habanero Chicken Wings

Prep:

20 mins

Cook:

1 hr 33 mins

Total:

1 hr 53 mins

Servings:

10

Yield:

30 wings

Ingredients

30 chicken wing sections
1 (12 ounce) can mango nectar
¼ cup brown sugar
6 habanero peppers, stemmed
2 tablespoons soy sauce
1 tablespoon sriracha hot chili sauce
1 tablespoon rice vinegar
1 stick butter
3 cloves garlic, minced
2 tablespoons honey
1 cup cornstarch
2 cups vegetable oil for frying

Directions

1

Rinse chicken wings and pat dry with paper towels. Place wings on a baking sheet and refrigerate to dry a bit more.

2

Combine mango nectar, brown sugar, habanero peppers, soy sauce, sriracha sauce, and vinegar in a food processor. Mix until peppers are pureed; seeds will still be visible. Remove food processor lid carefully; the pepper fumes can be strong.

3

Melt butter in a saucepan over medium heat. Add minced garlic; cook until fragrant, about 30 seconds. Add the mango-habanero mixture immediately; bring to a simmer, stirring frequently. Reduce heat to medium-low; add honey. Simmer, stirring frequently, until sauce is reduced by 75% and thickened to a glaze, 45 minutes to 1 hour. Remove from heat.

4

Preheat the oven to 200 degrees F (95 degrees C).

5

Heat oil in a deep-fryer to 350 degrees F (175 degrees C).

6

Coat wings lightly with cornstarch. Place 5 to 6 wings in the hot oil; fry until golden brown and crispy, about 8 minutes. Place wings on a paper towel to absorb excess oil; transfer to the preheated oven to keep warm. Repeat until all wings have been fried and drained.

7

Place wings in a large bowl. Pour half the sauce over the wings and mix, coating the wings with the sauce. Continue adding the remaining sauce until you have coated the wings to your liking.

Nutrition

Per Serving: 450 calories; protein 18.6g; carbohydrates 28.5g; fat 29g; cholesterol 80.3mg; sodium 366.6mg.

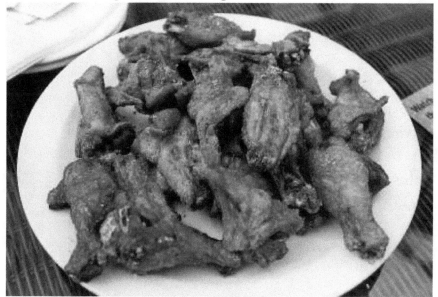

Italian Beef Ragout

Prep:

25 mins

Cook:

40 mins

Total:

1 hr 5 mins

Servings:

4

Yield:

4 Servings

Ingredients

¾ pound beef tenderloin, cut into 1/2 inch strips

1 tablespoon olive oil

1 ½ cups fresh mushrooms, sliced

1 medium onion, chopped

2 cloves garlic, minced

2 teaspoons all-purpose flour

½ teaspoon salt

¼ teaspoon black pepper

1 (14.5 ounce) can beef broth

¼ cup port wine

2 cups sugar snap peas

1 cup cherry tomatoes, cut in half

Directions

1

Heat olive oil in a large skillet over medium-high heat. Brown meat 2 to 3 minutes. Remove meat to paper towels. Stir in mushrooms, onion, and garlic; cook until onion is soft.

2

Sprinkle in flour, and stir well to mix. Season with salt and pepper. Stir in broth and wine; cook, stirring occasionally, until sauce is thickened. Stir in peas; cook 2 to 3 minutes more. Return meat to skillet. Stir in tomatoes, and heat through.

Nutrition

Per Serving: 367 calories; protein 20.4g; carbohydrates 15.1g; fat 23.5g; cholesterol 60.4mg; sodium 669.8mg.

Steak & Mushrooms

Prep:

15 mins

Cook:

25 mins

Total:

40 mins

Servings:

4

Yield:

4 servings

Ingredients

1 pound lean ground beef

⅓ cup dry bread crumbs

¼ cup chopped onions

1 egg, beaten

1 teaspoon salt

¼ teaspoon ground black pepper

2 cups beef broth

1 large onion, thinly sliced

1 cup sliced mushrooms

3 tablespoons cornstarch

3 tablespoons water

Directions

1

Combine ground beef, bread crumbs, chopped onion, egg, salt, and black pepper in a bowl until evenly mixed. Shape beef mixture into 4 patties, about 3/4 inch thick.

2

Fry patties in a large skillet over medium heat until browned on both sides, about 10 minutes. Add beef broth, onion, and mushrooms; bring to a boil. Reduce heat to low, cover, and simmer until patties are no longer pink in the center, about 10 minutes more. Transfer patties to a platter and keep warm.

3

Bring onion mixture to a boil. Mix cornstarch and water in a small bowl; stir into onion mixture. Cook and stir until onion gravy is thickened, about 1 minute. Pour over patties to serve.

Nutrition

Per Serving: 323 calories; protein 26.6g; carbohydrates 17.2g; fat 15.8g; cholesterol 115.3mg; sodium 1128.9mg.

Kale & Mushroom Galette

Prep:

20 mins

Cook:

15 mins

Total:

35 mins

Servings:

4

Yield:

4 servings

Ingredients

3 tablespoons butter

1 bunch kale, stems removed and leaves chopped

1 large shallot, thinly sliced

5 crimini mushrooms, sliced

¾ cup heavy whipping cream

¼ cup shredded Asiago cheese

4 cloves garlic, crushed to a paste

1 pinch salt and ground black pepper to taste

Directions

1

Heat butter in a large skillet over medium heat; cook and stir kale and shallot until kale is tender, about 5 minutes. Stir mushrooms, cream, Asiago cheese, garlic, salt, and black pepper into kale mixture. Reduce heat to low and simmer until cream has thickened and mushrooms are tender, about 10 minutes.

Nutrition

Per Serving: 333 calories; protein 7.9g; carbohydrates 16.7g; fat 27.9g; cholesterol 90.1mg; sodium 219.4mg.

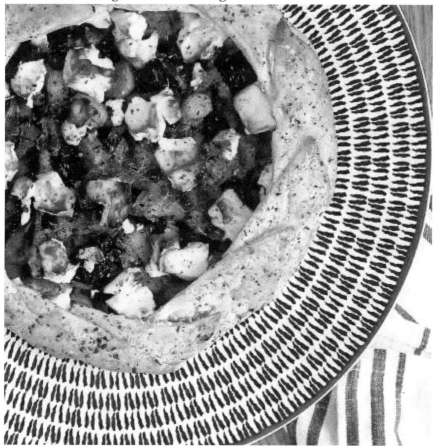

Meatless Meatballs

Prep:

15 mins

Cook:

1 hr 20 mins

Total:

1 hr 35 mins

Servings:

20

Yield:

100 small meatballs

Ingredients

4 cups shredded mozzarella cheese
8 eggs
2 cups cracker crumbs
1 ½ cups finely ground pecans
1 (1 ounce) package dry onion soup mix
2 teaspoons celery salt
vegetable oil for frying
1 (10.75 ounce) can condensed cream of mushroom soup
22 fluid ounces milk

Directions

1

Combine mozzarella cheese, eggs, cracker crumbs, pecans, onion soup mix, and celery salt in a large bowl. Form mixture into small meatballs.

2

Heat oil in a deep-fryer or large saucepan. Cook meatballs in batches until browned and crispy, about 5 minutes. Drain on a baking sheet lined paper towels.

3

Transfer meatballs to a large slow cooker. Cover with cream of mushroom soup. Use the empty can to measure and pour in milk. Cook on Low until flavors combine and soup mixture thickens, 30 minutes to 2 hours.

Nutrition

Per Serving: 246 calories; protein 11.1g; carbohydrates 14.4g; fat 16.3g; cholesterol 91.5mg; sodium 555.3mg.

Provolone Chicken Bake

Prep:

15 mins

Cook:

30 mins

Total:

45 mins

Servings:

8

Yield:

8 servings

Ingredients

8 skinless, boneless chicken breast halves

1 (16 ounce) package herb seasoned stuffing mix

2 (10.75 ounce) cans condensed cream of chicken soup

10 ¾ fluid ounces white wine

¼ cup melted butter

4 slices provolone cheese, halved

Directions

1

Preheat oven to 350 degrees F.

2

Arrange chicken breast halves in a single layer in a 9x13 inch baking dish. Top each breast half with a half slice of Provolone cheese.

3

In a medium bowl, blend cream of chicken soup and white wine. Pour over the chicken.

4

In a separate medium bowl, mix the butter and stuffing mix. Top the chicken with the stuffing mixture.

5

Bake 30 minutes in the preheated oven, or until chicken is no longer pink and juices run clear.

Nutrition

Per Serving: 555 calories; protein 39.3g; carbohydrates 49.8g; fat 17.3g; cholesterol 99.6mg; sodium 1524.7mg.

Prawn Saganaki

Prep:

15 mins

Cook:

35 mins

Total:

50 mins

Servings:

4

Yield:

4 servings

Ingredients

1 tablespoon olive oil

3 cloves garlic, thinly sliced

2 tablespoons tomato paste

1 ½ pounds prawns, peeled and deveined, tail on

½ cup white wine

1 (13.5 ounce) jar tomato and olive pasta sauce (such as Papayiannides® Tomato & Olive & Ouzo Sauce)

½ cup crumbled Greek feta cheese

2 tablespoons chopped fresh flat-leaf parsley

1 red onion, halved and thinly sliced

Directions

1

Preheat oven to 400 degrees F.

2

Heat olive oil in a large skillet over medium heat; cook and stir onion until soft, about 5 minutes. Stir in garlic and cook until fragrant, about 1 minute. Stir tomato paste into onion mixture; cook and stir for 1 minute.

3

Pour wine into tomato mixture; simmer until liquid is reduced by about half, about 5 minutes. Stir tomato sauce into wine mixture and simmer until mixture is thick, about 10 minutes.

4

Spread tomato mixture into the base of a 6-cup baking dish; top with prawns and sprinkle evenly with feta cheese.

5

Bake in the preheated oven until prawns are bright pink on the outside and the meat is no longer transparent in the center, about 10 minutes; top with parsley.

Nutrition

Per Serving: 341 calories; protein 33g; carbohydrates 19.7g; fat 11.5g; cholesterol 277.5mg; sodium 967.5mg.

Cauliflower Rice

Prep:

10 mins

Cook:

20 mins

Total:

30 mins

Servings:

4

Yield:

4 servings

Ingredients

1 head cauliflower, cut into florets

2 teaspoons chopped fresh chives

¼ teaspoon garlic powder

2 teaspoons chopped fresh parsley

salt and ground black pepper to taste

¼ teaspoon onion powder

Directions

1

Place a steamer insert into a pot and fill with water to just below the bottom of the steamer. Bring water to a boil. Add cauliflower, cover, and steam until fork-tender, 10 to 15 minutes.

2

Remove cauliflower and steamer from the pot. Drain all water and return cauliflower to the empty pot. Add chives, parsley, garlic powder, and onion powder.

3

Set pot over medium-low heat. Mash cauliflower with a potato masher to the consistency of rice grains. Stir until excess moisture evaporates and the 'rice' appears fluffy, 6 to 7 minutes. Season with salt and pepper.

Nutrition

Per Serving: 37 calories; protein 2.9g; carbohydrates 7.9g; fat 0.2g; sodium 82.4mg.

CHAPTER 5: **APPETIZER, SNACKS & SIDE DISHES**

Grilled Portobello Mushrooms

Prep:

10 mins

Cook:

10 mins

Additional:

1 hr

Total:

1 hr 20 mins

Servings:

3

Yield:

3 servings

Ingredients

3 mushrooms portobello mushrooms

¼ cup canola oil

3 tablespoons chopped onion

4 cloves garlic, minced

4 tablespoons balsamic vinegar

Directions

1

Clean mushrooms and remove stems, reserve for other use. Place caps on a plate with the gills up.

2

In a small bowl, combine the oil, onion, garlic and vinegar. Pour mixture evenly over the mushroom caps and let stand for 1 hour.

3

Grill over hot grill for 10 minutes. Serve immediately.

Nutrition

Per Serving: 217 calories; protein 3.2g; carbohydrates 11g; fat 19g; sodium 12.9mg.

Jalapeno Nacho with Shrimps

Prep:

20 mins

Cook:

5 mins

Total:

25 mins

Servings:

15

Yield:

50 nachos

Ingredients

½ cup sour cream
½ avocado, peeled and pitted
½ lemon, juiced
1 pound small Gulf shrimp (50 to 60 per pound), thawed and drained
1 tablespoon vegetable oil
¼ teaspoon ground dried chipotle pepper
salt and ground black pepper to taste
1 pinch cayenne pepper, or to taste
50 large (restaurant-style) tortilla chips, or as needed
2 jalapeno peppers, seeded and very thinly sliced
3 ½ cups shredded pepperjack cheese, or as needed
15 cherry tomatoes, sliced - or as needed
¼ cup chopped fresh cilantro

Directions

1

Combine sour cream, avocado, and lemon juice in a blender or food processor; blend until smooth and creamy. Transfer into a plastic decorating bottle with a long tip. Refrigerate avocado-cream sauce until needed.

2

Place shrimp into a bowl; combine with vegetable oil, ground chipotle pepper, salt, black pepper, and cayenne pepper.

3

Place a large nonstick pan over high heat. Cook shrimp in the hot pan in a single layer until barely cooked through and pink, about 1 minute per side. Transfer to a plate and let shrimp cool.

4

Preheat the oven's broiler. Line a baking sheet with aluminum foil and lightly grease the foil.

5

Lay tortilla chips onto the prepared baking sheet in a single layer. Place 1 shrimp onto each chip. Add 1 slice jalapeno and 1 large pinch pepperjack cheese on top of each shrimp.

6

Broil under preheated broiler until cheese is melted and chips are lightly toasted, about 1 minute. Watch carefully; chips will burn quickly.

7

Remove nachos from baking sheet and arrange onto a serving platter; drizzle with avocado-cream sauce and sprinkle with cherry tomatoes and cilantro before serving.

Nutrition

Per Serving: 209 calories; protein 12.5g; carbohydrates 6.3g; fat 14.9g; cholesterol 82.4mg; sodium 277.7mg.

Chicken Paprika

Prep:

20 mins

Cook:

20 mins

Total:

40 mins

Servings:

12

Yield:

12 servings

Ingredients

⅓ cup all-purpose flour

2 tablespoons paprika

1 teaspoon salt

1 pinch ground black pepper

6 skinless, boneless chicken breast halves, cut into bite-size pieces

2 tablespoons vegetable oil

1 onion, chopped

4 cloves garlic, minced

1 cup chicken stock

2 tablespoons tomato paste

1 ½ cups sour cream

1 tablespoon paprika

1 teaspoon cornstarch

Directions

1

Mix flour, 2 tablespoons paprika, salt, and pepper on a shallow plate.
Dip chicken pieces in mixture to coat.

2

Heat vegetable oil in a heavy skillet over medium heat. Cook and stir
chicken in hot oil until browned completely, about 5 minutes. Remove
chicken with a slotted spoon to a bowl, reserving oil and drippings in
skillet.

3

Cook and stir onion and garlic in the reserved drippings until tender,
about 5 minutes. Return chicken to the skillet. Pour chicken stock over
the chicken mixture. Stir tomato paste into the chicken stock until
integrated completely.

4

Bring the chicken stock to a boil, reduce heat to medium-low, place a
cover on the skillet, and cook at a simmer until the chicken is cooked
through, 5 to 8 minutes.

5

Whisk sour cream, 1 teaspoon paprika, and cornstarch together in a
small bowl; stir into the chicken mixture and cook until hot, 2 to 3
minutes.

Nutrition

Per Serving: 170 calories; protein 13g; carbohydrates 7.8g; fat 9.8g;
cholesterol 42mg; sodium 313.1mg.

CHAPTER 6: VEGAN & VEGETARIAN

Greek Pizza with Spinach, Feta and Olives

Prep:

30 mins

Cook:

12 mins

Total:

42 mins

Servings:

6

Yield:

6 slices

Ingredients

½ cup mayonnaise

2 cups baby spinach leaves

1 cup crumbled feta cheese, divided

1 (12 inch) pre-baked Italian pizza crust

½ cup oil-packed sun-dried tomatoes, coarsely chopped

1 tablespoon oil from the sun-dried tomatoes

4 cloves garlic, minced

¼ cup pitted kalamata olives, coarsely chopped

1 teaspoon dried oregano

½ small red onion, halved and thinly sliced

Directions

1

Adjust oven rack to lowest position, and heat oven to 450 degrees. Mix mayonnaise, garlic and 1/2 cup feta in a small bowl. Place pizza crust on a cookie sheet; spread mayonnaise mixture over pizza, then top with tomatoes, olives and oregano. Bake until heated through and crisp, about 10 minutes.

2

Toss spinach and onion with the 1 Tb. sun-dried tomato oil. Top hot pizza with spinach mixture and remaining 1/2 cup feta cheese. Return to oven and bake until cheese melts, about 2 minutes longer. Cut into 6 slices and serve.

Nutrition

Per Serving: 461 calories; protein 14.1g; carbohydrates 39.3g; fat 29g; cholesterol 35.9mg; sodium 894.4mg.

Stuffed Portobello Mushrooms

Prep:

15 mins

Cook:

20 mins

Total:

35 mins

Servings:

4

Yield:

4 servings

Ingredients

½ cup finely chopped red bell pepper

¼ cup olive oil

4 portobello mushroom caps

¼ teaspoon onion powder

1 teaspoon salt

½ teaspoon ground black pepper

1 clove garlic, minced

Directions

1

Preheat grill for medium heat.

2

In a large bowl, mix the red bell pepper, garlic, oil, onion powder, salt, and ground black pepper. Spread mixture over gill side of the mushroom caps.

3

Lightly oil the grill grate. Place mushrooms over indirect heat, cover, and cook for 15 to 20 minutes.

Nutrition

Per Serving: 157 calories; protein 3.1g; carbohydrates 7.3g; fat 13.8g; sodium 589.4mg.

Brussels Sprouts Caesar

Prep:

20 mins

Cook:

20 mins

Total:

40 mins

Servings:

6

Yield:

6 servings

Ingredients

2 (16 ounce) packages Brussels sprouts

¼ cup olive oil, divided

2 teaspoons smoked paprika, divided

¼ teaspoon sea salt

¼ cup heavy whipping cream

1 tablespoon red wine vinegar

1 lemon, zested and juiced

2 cloves garlic, minced

1 teaspoon brown mustard

3 tablespoons grated Parmesan cheese

Directions

1

Preheat oven to 425 degrees F.

2

Trim stems off Brussels sprouts. Quarter large sprouts lengthwise; halve small ones. Rinse and dry completely.

3

Toss sprouts in a bowl with 1 tablespoon olive oil and 1 teaspoon paprika. Spread out on a baking sheet and sprinkle with sea salt.

4

Bake in the preheated oven for 20 minutes, removing loose leaves after 5 minutes and turning whole sprouts every 5 minutes.

5

Whisk remaining 3 tablespoons olive oil, remaining 1 teaspoon paprika, heavy cream, Parmesan cheese, red wine vinegar, lemon zest and juice, garlic, and brown mustard together in a bowl.

6

Transfer whole sprouts and any loose leaves to a bowl; pour in cream mixture and toss to combine.

Nutrition

Per Serving: 199 calories; protein 6.7g; carbohydrates 16.9g; fat 14g; cholesterol 15.8mg; sodium 165.1mg.

Vegetarian Meatballs

Prep:

15 mins

Cook:

1 hr 20 mins

Total:

1 hr 35 mins

Servings:

20

Yield:

100 small meatballs

Ingredients

4 cups shredded mozzarella cheese

1 ½ cups finely ground pecans

1 (1 ounce) package dry onion soup mix

22 fluid ounces milk

2 teaspoons celery salt

8 eggs

2 cups cracker crumbs

vegetable oil for frying

1 (10.75 ounce) can condensed cream of mushroom soup

Directions

1

Combine mozzarella cheese, eggs, cracker crumbs, pecans, onion soup mix, and celery salt in a large bowl. Form mixture into small meatballs.

2

Heat oil in a deep-fryer or large saucepan. Cook meatballs in batches until browned and crispy, about 5 minutes. Drain on a baking sheet lined paper towels.

3

Transfer meatballs to a large slow cooker. Cover with cream of mushroom soup. Use the empty can to measure and pour in milk. Cook on Low until flavors combine and soup mixture thickens, 30 minutes to 2 hours.

Nutrition

Per Serving: 246 calories; protein 11.1g; carbohydrates 14.4g; fat 16.3g; cholesterol 91.5mg; sodium 555.3mg.

Dal Makhani (Indian Lentils)

Prep:

15 mins

Cook:

2 hrs

Additional:

2 hrs

Total:

4 hrs 15 mins

Servings:

6

Yield:

6 servings

Ingredients

1 cup lentils

water to cover

5 cups water

salt to taste

2 tablespoons vegetable oil

1 tablespoon cumin seeds

4 cardamom pods

4 bay leaves

6 whole cloves

1 ½ tablespoons ginger paste

½ teaspoon ground turmeric

1 ½ tablespoons garlic paste

1 cinnamon stick, broken

1 pinch cayenne pepper

1 cup canned tomato puree, or more to taste

2 tablespoons ground coriander

¼ cup butter

1 tablespoon chili powder

Directions

1

Place lentils and kidney beans in a large bowl; cover with plenty of water. Soak for at least 2 hours or overnight. Drain.

2

Cook lentils, kidney beans, 5 cups water, and salt in a pot over medium heat until tender, stirring occasionally, about 1 hour. Remove from heat and set aside. Keep the lentils, kidney beans, and any excess cooking water in the pot.

3

Heat vegetable oil in a saucepan over medium-high heat. Cook cumin seeds in the hot oil until they begin to pop, 1 to 2 minutes. Add cardamom pods, cinnamon stick, bay leaves, and cloves; cook until bay leaves turn brown, about 1 minute. Reduce heat to medium-low; add ginger paste, garlic paste, turmeric, and cayenne pepper. Stir to coat.

4

Stir tomato puree into spice mixture; cook over medium heat until slightly reduced, about 5 minutes. Add chili powder, coriander, and butter; cook and stir until butter is melted.

5

Stir lentils, kidney beans and any leftover cooking water into tomato mixture; bring to a boil, reduce heat to low. Stir fenugreek into lentil mixture. Cover saucepan and simmer until heated through, stirring occasionally, about 45 minutes. Add cream and cook until heated through, 2 to 4 minutes.

Nutrition

Per Serving: 390 calories; protein 13.2g; carbohydrates 37.1g; fat 21.5g; cholesterol 47.5mg; sodium 420.2mg.

CHAPTER 7: DESSERTS

Chocolate Ice Cream

Prep:

20 mins

Additional:

6 hrs

Total:

6 hrs 20 mins

Servings:

12

Yield:

1 - 9x5 loaf

Ingredients

1 (14 ounce) can sweetened condensed milk

2 cups heavy cream

⅔ cup chocolate syrup

Directions

1

Line a 9x5 inch loaf pan with aluminum foil. In a large bowl, stir together condensed milk and chocolate syrup until color is even. In a separate bowl, whip cream until stiff peaks form. Fold cream into chocolate mixture and pour all into prepared pan. Cover and freeze 6 hours, until firm.

Nutrition

Per Serving: 288 calories; protein 3.7g; carbohydrates 29.7g; fat 17.7g; cholesterol 65.5mg; sodium 68.6mg.

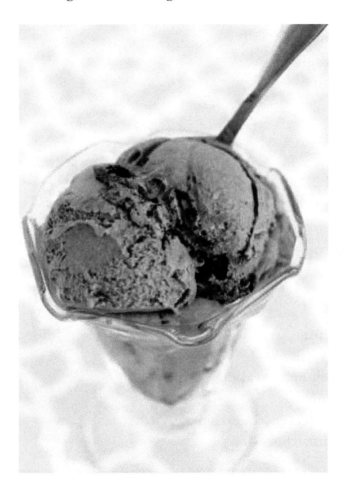

Chocolate Pudding

Prep:

5 mins

Cook:

15 mins

Additional:

3 hrs

Total:

3 hrs 20 mins

Servings:

6

Yield:

6 servings

Ingredients

3 cups whole milk, divided

⅓ cup white sugar

1 cup semisweet chocolate chips

¼ cup cornstarch

Directions

1

Combine 1/2 cup milk and cornstarch in a small bowl. Whisk or stir with a fork until smooth and all lumps have been incorporated.

2

Combine remaining milk with sugar in a medium saucepan over low heat. Slowly whisk in the cornstarch mixture. Cook, whisking as needed to prevent lumps from forming, until mixture begins to thicken, 8 to 10 minutes. Add chocolate chips and salt. Continue stirring until chips are completely melted and pudding is smooth and thickened, about 8 minutes more.

3

Pour pudding into 1 large bowl or 6 individual bowls. Place plastic wrap directly on top of the pudding to prevent a skin from forming; smooth it gently against the surface. Refrigerate for at least 3 to 4 hours before serving.

Nutrition

Per Serving: 271 calories; protein 5.1g; carbohydrates 39.2g; fat 12.4g; cholesterol 12.2mg; sodium 78.2mg.

Frozen Banana Bites

Prep:

30 mins

Cook:

1 hr 45 mins

Total:

2 hrs 15 mins

Servings:

48

Yield:

48 servings

Ingredients

1 cup peanut butter

4 bananas, sliced into 1-inch rounds

1 tablespoon shortening

⅓ cup toffee baking bits

8 (1 ounce) squares semisweet chocolate

Directions

1

Cover a baking sheet with waxed paper.

2

Spoon a thin layer of peanut butter on top of each banana slice. Insert a toothpick through the peanut butter layer into the banana. Place banana bites onto the prepared baking sheet; freeze for 30 minutes to overnight.

3

Melt chocolate and shortening in the top of a double boiler over simmering water, stirring frequently and scraping down the sides with a rubber spatula to avoid scorching.

4

Cover another baking sheet with waxed paper.

5

Remove 2 to 4 banana bites from the freezer at a time; coat each bite with chocolate mixture. Place coated banana bites on the second baking sheet; sprinkle each with toffee bits. Repeat until all the bites are coated. Return banana bites to freezer until set, at least 1 hour. Allow bites to sit in room temperature for about 15 minutes before serving.

Nutrition

Per Serving: 76 calories; protein 1.8g; carbohydrates 6.9g; fat 5.1g; cholesterol 1.4mg; sodium 32.9mg.

Mocha Mousse Cups

Prep:

4 mins

Cook:

1 min

Total:

5 mins

Servings:

1

Yield:

1 serving

Ingredients

1 ¼ cups 2% milk
1 (1.5 fluid ounce) jigger brewed espresso
2 tablespoons chocolate syrup

Directions

1

Pour milk into a steaming pitcher and heat to 145 degrees F to 165 degrees F using the steaming wand. Measure the chocolate syrup into a large coffee mug. Brew espresso, then add to mug. Pour the steamed milk into the mug, using a spoon to hold back the foam. Top with whipped cream.

Nutrition

Per Serving: 266 calories; protein 11g; carbohydrates 39.1g; fat 7.2g; cholesterol 26.7mg; sodium 162mg.

Caramel Cake

Prep:

40 mins

Cook:

37 mins

Additional:

1 hr 5 mins

Total:

2 hrs 22 mins

Servings:

12

Yield:

1 9-inch layer cake

Ingredients

Cake:

3 cups white sugar

1 ½ cups butter

½ teaspoon baking powder

¼ teaspoon salt

5 eggs

3 ½ cups all-purpose flour

1 ¼ cups whole milk

1 teaspoon vanilla extract

Icing:

1 (16 ounce) package brown sugar

¼ teaspoon salt

⅔ cup evaporated milk

1 cup butter

1 (16 ounce) package confectioners' sugar, sifted
2 teaspoons pure vanilla extract

Directions

1

Preheat oven to 350 degrees F. Grease and flour three 9-inch cake pans.

2

Cream white sugar, 1 1/2 cups butter, and eggs together in a bowl. Beat well.

3

Combine flour, baking powder, and 1/4 teaspoon salt. Add to the sugar mixture alternately with milk. Add vanilla extract. Beat until batter makes ribbons when falling from the whisk or beater. Divide batter among the prepared cake pans.

4

Bake in the preheated oven until a toothpick inserted in the center comes out clean, about 30 minutes. Cool layers on a rack before icing, at least 1 hour.

5

Combine brown sugar, 1 cup butter, and 1/4 teaspoon salt in a saucepan over medium heat. Stir until brown sugar is dissolved, about 3 minutes. Add evaporated milk and continue stirring. Bring to a gentle boil and let bubble for about 4 minutes, stirring constantly to avoid sticking. Remove from heat and allow to cool, about 5 minutes.

6

Mix confectioners' sugar and vanilla extract into the butter-milk mixture using an electric mixer until icing caramelizes and thickens to the desired consistency.

7

Spread icing onto the cooled cake layers. Stack layers; ice top and sides.

Nutrition

Per Serving: 1019 calories; protein 8.6g; carbohydrates 154.5g; fat 42.7g; cholesterol 185.8mg; sodium 455.4mg.

Blueberry Pecan Crisp

Prep:

15 mins

Cook:

40 mins

Total:

55 mins

Servings:

8

Yield:

8 servings

Ingredients

1 ½ cups all-purpose flour

¾ cup brown sugar

1 cup white sugar

¼ cup orange juice

2 tablespoons instant tapioca

1 teaspoon cinnamon

½ cup cold butter, diced

½ teaspoon salt

6 cups fresh blueberries

Directions

1

Preheat oven to 375 degrees F.

2

Combine flour, brown sugar, butter, and salt in food processor; pulse mixture into coarse crumbs.

3

Stir sugar, orange juice, tapioca, and cinnamon together in a bowl; add blueberries and stir to coat completely. Spoon blueberry mixture into a large baking dish. Sprinkle crumbs over the blueberries.

4

Bake in preheated oven until topping is golden brown and the filling bubbles, about 40 minutes.

Nutrition

Per Serving: 398 calories; protein 3.3g; carbohydrates 74.1g; fat 11.9g; cholesterol 30.5mg; sodium 232.1mg.

Classic Candied Sweet Potatoes

Prep:

15 mins

Cook:

1 hr 35 mins

Total:

1 hr 50 mins

Servings:

8

Yield:

8 servings

Ingredients

½ cup butter

½ cup water

1 teaspoon salt

1 cup packed brown sugar

6 yellow-fleshed sweet potatoes

Directions

1

Preheat oven to 350 degrees F.

2

Place whole sweet potatoes in a steamer over a couple of inches of boiling water, and cover. Cook until tender, about 30 minutes. Drain and cool.

3

Peel, and slice sweet potatoes lengthwise into 1/2 inch slices. Place in a 9x13 inch baking dish.

4

In a small saucepan over medium heat, melt butter, brown sugar, water and salt. When the sauce is bubbly and sugar is dissolved, pour over potatoes.

5

Bake in preheated oven for 1 hour, occasionally basting the sweet potatoes with the brown sugar sauce.

Nutrition

Per Serving: 294 calories; protein 2.1g; carbohydrates 47.2g; fat 11.7g; cholesterol 30.5mg; sodium 415.2mg.

Keto Donuts

Prep:

20 mins

Cook:

20 mins

Additional:

5 mins

Total:

45 mins

Servings:

12

Yield:

12 donuts

Ingredients

baking spray
2 cups all-purpose flour
1 ¼ cups white sugar
2 teaspoons baking powder
½ teaspoon pumpkin pie spice
½ teaspoon kosher salt
1 cup applesauce
1 teaspoon ground cinnamon
1 cup apple cider
1 extra large egg, lightly beaten
2 teaspoons vanilla extract
2 tablespoons unsalted butter, melted
Topping:
½ cup white sugar

4 tablespoons unsalted butter, melted

½ teaspoon ground cinnamon

Directions

1

Preheat the oven to 350 degrees F. Spray a 12-cup muffin pan with baking spray.

2

Sift flour, sugar, baking powder, cinnamon, pumpkin pie spice, and kosher salt together in a bowl.

3

Whisk applesauce, apple cider, melted butter, egg, and vanilla extract together in a small bowl. Stir into flour mixture gradually until **Ingredients** are combined.

4

Spoon batter into the prepared pan, filling each cup 3/4 full.

5

Bake in the preheated oven until a toothpick inserted into the center of a donut comes out clean, about 17 minutes. Remove from the oven and let cool for 5 minutes before removing donuts from the pan.

6

Combine sugar and cinnamon for topping in a shallow dish. Brush donuts with melted butter on both sides and dip into sugar-cinnamon combination.

Nutrition

Per Serving: 270 calories; protein 2.9g; carbohydrates 50.7g; fat 6.5g; cholesterol 33.2mg; sodium 172.1mg.

Minty Cookies

Prep:

20 mins

Cook:

10 mins

Additional:

20 mins

Total:

50 mins

Servings:

35

Yield:

35 cookies

Ingredients

1 cup butter, softened

½ cup cocoa powder

1 teaspoon baking soda

1 cup white sugar

¾ cup packed light brown sugar

2 teaspoons vanilla extract

½ teaspoon salt

2 eggs

1 tablespoon peppermint extract

2 cups all-purpose flour

1 ⅔ cups mint chocolate chips

Directions

1

Preheat oven to 375 degrees F.

2

Beat butter, white sugar, brown sugar, peppermint extract, vanilla extract, and salt together in a bowl using an electric mixer until smooth and creamy. Beat eggs into butter mixture until well incorporated.

3

Whisk flour, cocoa powder, and baking soda together in a bowl; gradually add to creamed butter mixture, beating until dough is well blended. Fold chocolate chips into dough. Drop dough by rounded teaspoons onto a baking sheet.

4

Bake in the preheated oven until cookies are set in the middle, 8 to 10 minutes. Cool cookies on the baking sheet for about 5 minutes before transferring to a wire rack to cool completely.

Nutrition

Per Serving: 161 calories; protein 2g; carbohydrates 21.6g; fat 8g; cholesterol 24.6mg; sodium 112.3mg.

Cinnamon-Caramel-Nut Rolls

Prep:

20 mins

Cook:

36 mins

Additional:

1 hr 5 mins

Total:

2 hrs 1 min

Servings:

14

Yield:

1 9x13-inch pan

Ingredients

1 cup chopped walnuts

2 (1 pound) loaves frozen bread dough, thawed

1 cup brown sugar

1 (5.1 ounce) package non-instant vanilla pudding mix

½ cup butter

2 teaspoons milk

Directions

1

Grease a 9x13-inch baking pan and sprinkle the bottom with walnuts. Tear thawed dough into pieces and place into the pan.

2

Combine brown sugar, pudding mix, butter, 3 teaspoons cinnamon, and milk in a saucepan. Cook over low heat until dissolved, 6 to 8 minutes. Pour over the dough. Sprinkle with 1 teaspoon cinnamon. Cover rolls with a clean kitchen towel and let rise until doubled in size, 1 to 2 hours.

3

Preheat oven to 350 degrees F.

4

Bake rolls in the preheated oven until golden brown, about 30 minutes.

5

Allow to cool, about 5 minutes. Flip rolls out of pan and serve warm.

Nutrition

Per Serving: 396 calories; protein 7.9g; carbohydrates 57.9g; fat 14.8g; cholesterol 17.4mg; sodium 492.4mg.

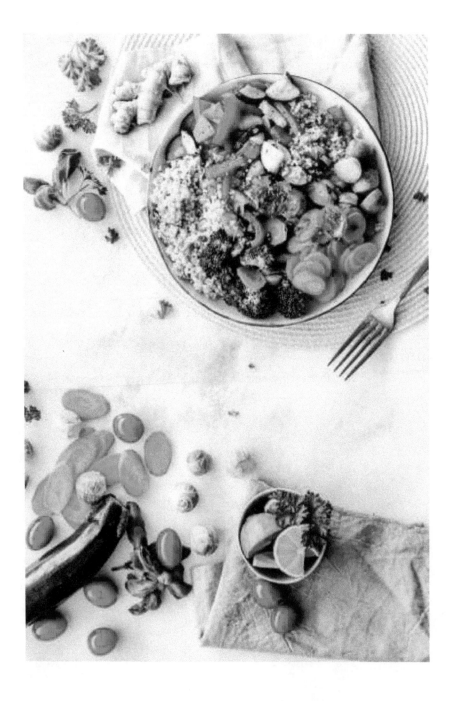